Table of Contents

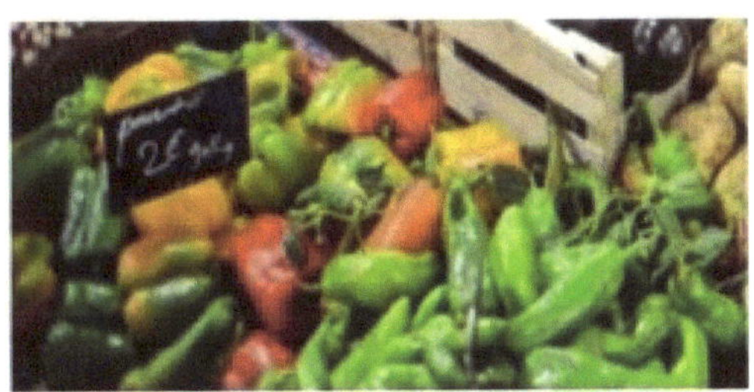

When we talk about the ketogenic diet many question arise. In some cases it can be confusing. These keto-related questions might arise from a person who wants to start a ketogenic diet for the first time.

We have compiled information related to the Keto Diet and answers to the comprehensive list of questions above. It is recommended you read this book as a starting point to get information if you're new to Keto. Use the Keto Meal Plan and recipes in this book as part of your diet plan. After reading this book, you will understand how to enter the ketosis phase quickly and lose a few pounds within a week after starting the Keto Diet.

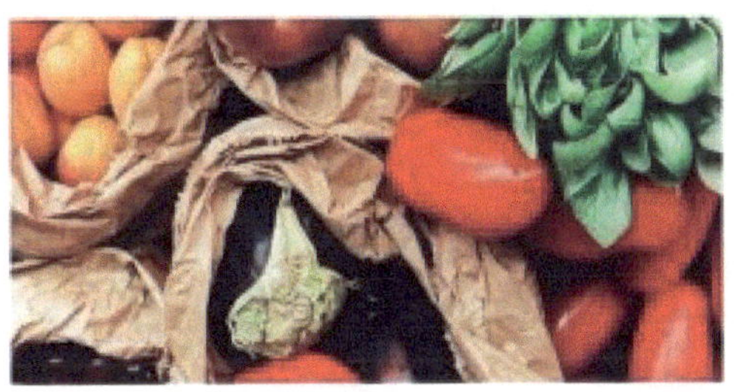

Easy Keto Diet
By Lyndi Kae

FACEBOOK: @ForYouABetterLife

Email address: foryouabetterlife@gmail.com

Website: https://for-yous.com

Original Edition

Copyright © 2020 by Publisher:

Sweetwater Publishing Company

6612 Ky. Hwy. 17 North, DeMossville, KY 41033

www.sweetwaterpublishingcompany.wordpress.com

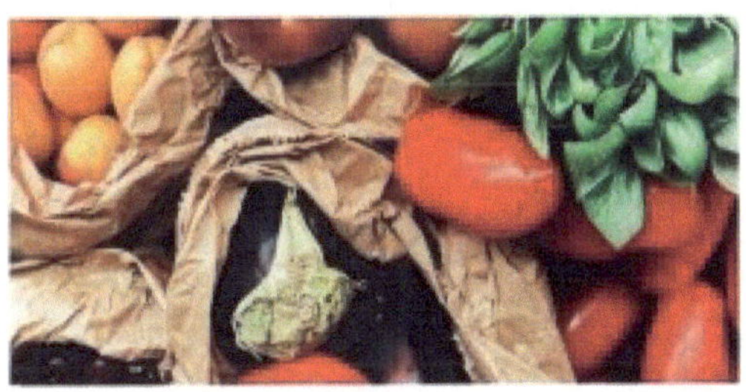

THE SCIENCE

A study by Harvard University shows that eating highly processed foods like fast food or candy bars cause the brain to release a blast of chemicals like dopamine and serotonin, providing a feel-good rush. Like drugs such as cocaine, the brain becomes trained from sugar, and it forms an addiction of sorts. The brain forgets how to produce these happy chemicals in a healthy manner. The body craves it more and more. The rush wanes with further consumption, so it takes more to get that same feel-good sensation as the body develops a tolerance for it. Indulgence results in weight gain.

BREAK THE CYCLE

Your Ketosis Diet eliminates sugar and unhealthy fat culprits causing the problem. Your healthy eating plan nurtures your body and retrains your brain to produce serotonin and dopamine naturally.

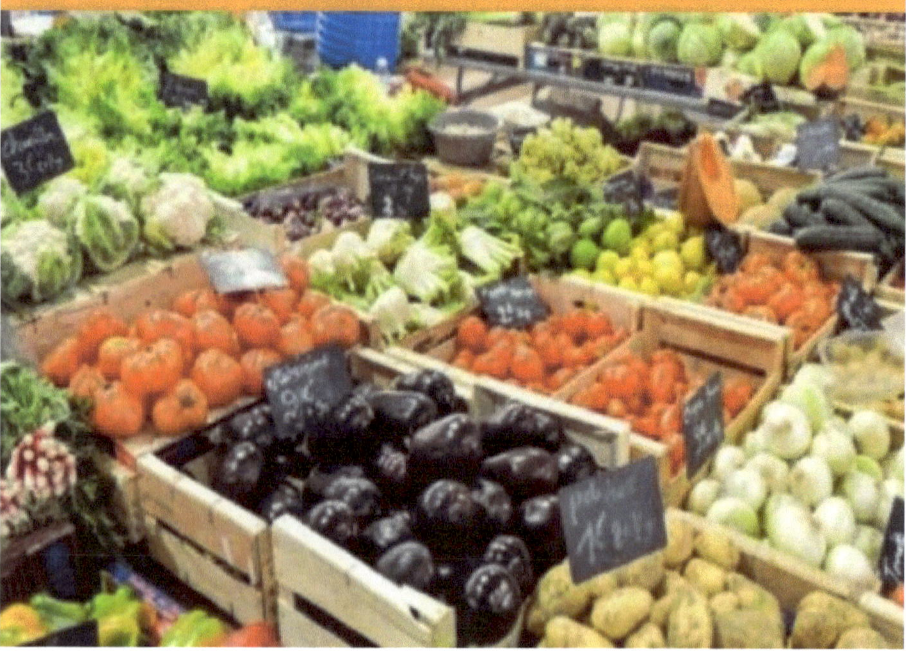

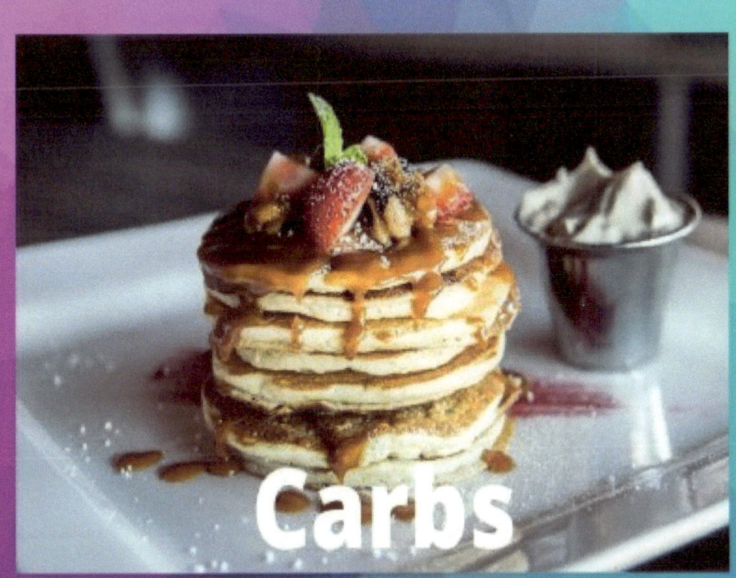

The most crucial factor in achieving ketosis is eating a very low-carbohydrate diet.

Your body cells usually burn glucose or sugar as their principal fuel source. Most cells can, however, use other fuels like fatty acids and ketones, also known as ketone bodies.

The body holds glucose in the form of glycogen. Glycogen storage is reduced. Hormone insulin levels decline when carb intake is very low. This allows release of fatty acids from your body's fatty stores.

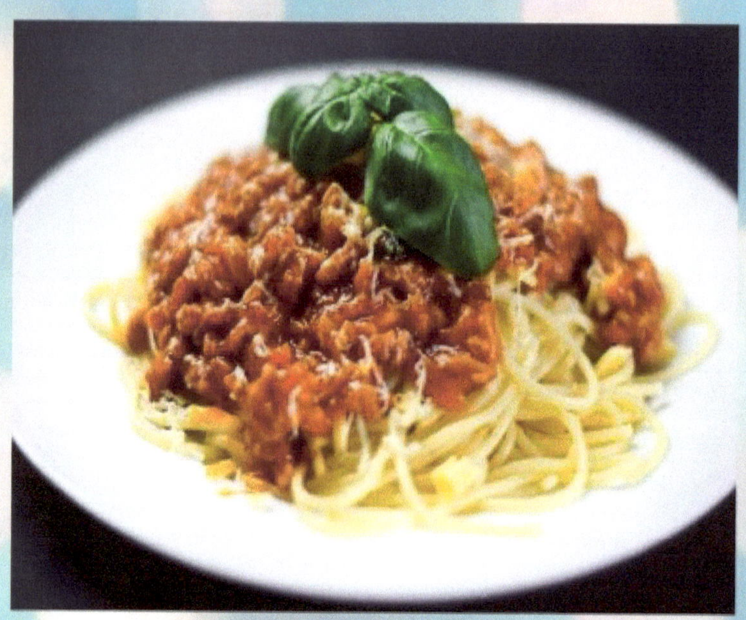

Some fatty acids in your liver are converted to ketones, acetone and beta-hydroxybutyrate. Sections of the brain use ketones as a source of energy.

Carb restriction to induce ketosis varies by individuals. Many people can achieve ketosis with net carbohydrates of 20 grams a day. Others can reach ketosis by consuming twice or more. The range is generally between 20-50 grams per day in order for most people to achieve ketosis.

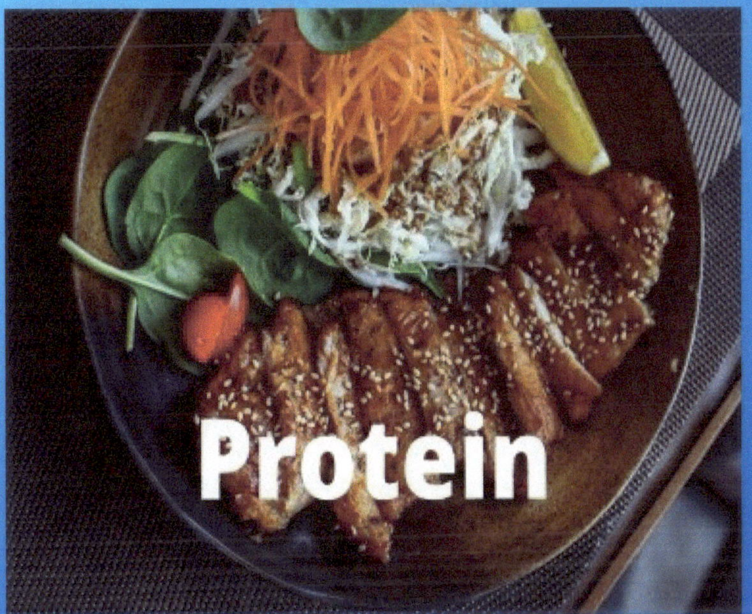

Maintain enough protein consumption. Achieving ketosis requires an adequate but not excessive intake of protein.

Ketogenic Diets lead to increased intake of protein, which provides numerous weight loss benefits, and restricts intake of carbahydrates. This substantially decreases calorie intake, which is necessary for weight loss without counting calories.

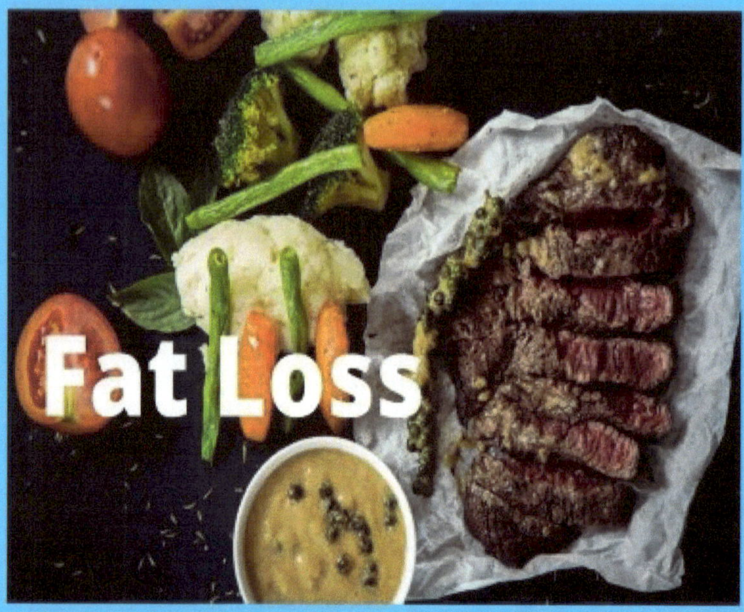

Your abdominal cavity produces a higher proportion of fat loss with help of a Keto Diet. Not all fat is the same in your body. When fat is processed, it determines how it impacts your health and disease risk.

The two main types are subcutaneous fat under your skin and visceral fat accumulated in your abdominal cavity. Visceral fat sits around the liver. Excess visceral fat is linked to inflammation and resistance to insulin—and can cause today's western metabolic dysfunction. Low-carb diets reduce this harmful abdominal fat extremely efficiently.

"EARLY RESULTS"
"NO CALORIE COUNTING"

You begin to prefer healthy foods. Brain fog vanishes. Energy intensifies. You lose weight and transform your life dramatically. Results are evident quickly and bolsters your determination to stick it out, because you see early signs it's working for you.

There's no calorie counting. You shed weight through ketosis.

"YOUR BODY BECOMES A FAT-BURNING MACHINE"

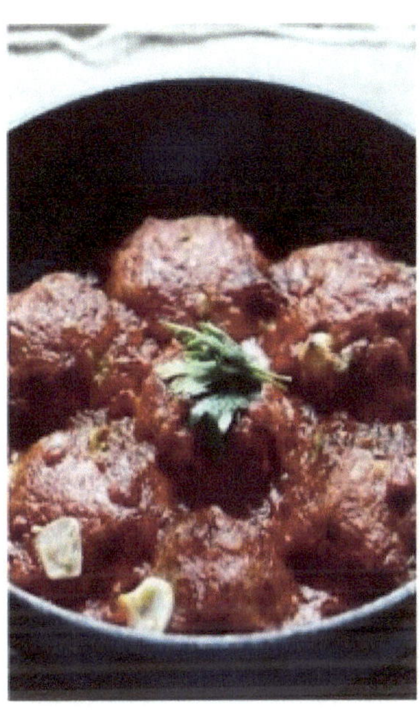

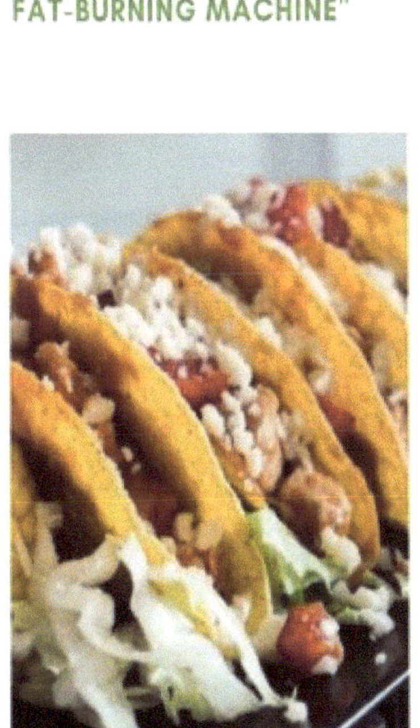

WHAT IS KETOSIS?

The body generates ketones as a source of energy when you limit carbohydrate consumption. Ketones are made of the fatty acids found in food or body fat in your liver. The liver uses fat to produce ketones. Thus, instead of carbohydrates, ketones are used for energy production. When your body continuously consumes fat as a source of food and you have reduced carbohydrate intake, you lose body fat and weight.

Because your body in ketosis burns fat for fuel, you might think keto can work on specific problem areas, such as belly fat. Burning belly fat is high on the priority list of many people. This dangerous fat inside your abdomen surrounds your organs and is associated with heart disease and diabetes type 2.

The Keto Diet automatically spot-targets fat reduction areas. Your body decides where the weight loss takes place.

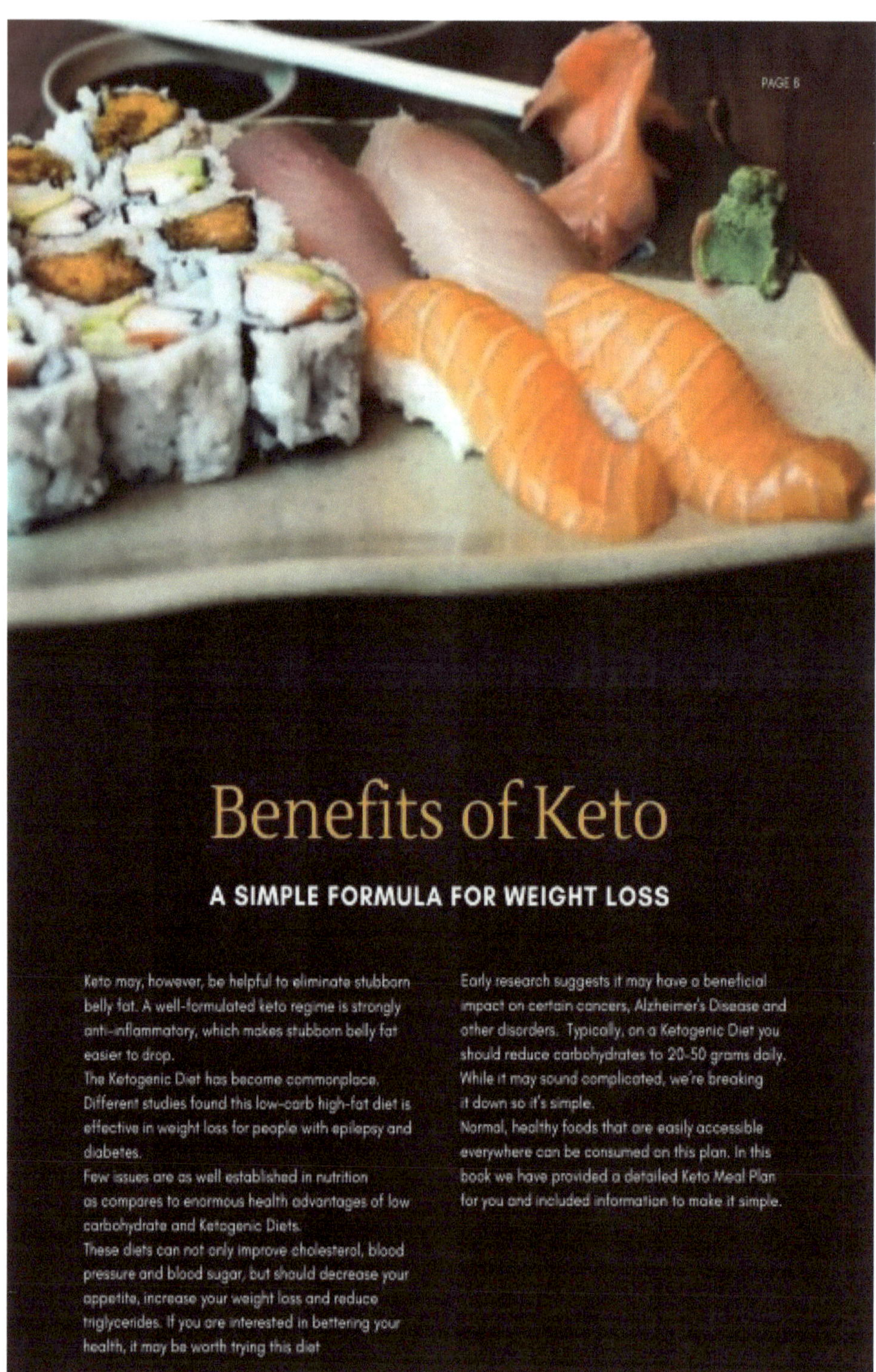

Benefits of Keto

A SIMPLE FORMULA FOR WEIGHT LOSS

Keto may, however, be helpful to eliminate stubborn belly fat. A well-formulated keto regime is strongly anti-inflammatory, which makes stubborn belly fat easier to drop.

The Ketogenic Diet has become commonplace. Different studies found this low-carb high-fat diet is effective in weight loss for people with epilepsy and diabetes.

Few issues are as well established in nutrition as compares to enormous health advantages of low carbohydrate and Ketogenic Diets.

These diets can not only improve cholesterol, blood pressure and blood sugar, but should decrease your appetite, increase your weight loss and reduce triglycerides. If you are interested in bettering your health, it may be worth trying this diet

Early research suggests it may have a beneficial impact on certain cancers, Alzheimer's Disease and other disorders. Typically, on a Ketogenic Diet you should reduce carbohydrates to 20-50 grams daily. While it may sound complicated, we're breaking it down so it's simple.

Normal, healthy foods that are easily accessible everywhere can be consumed on this plan. In this book we have provided a detailed Keto Meal Plan for you and included information to make it simple.

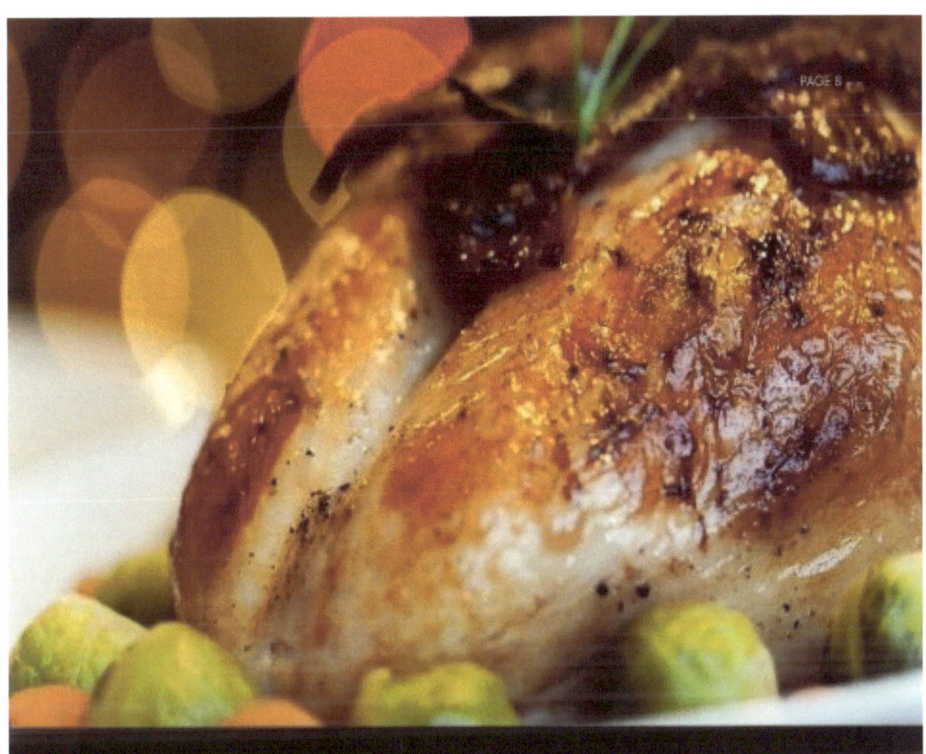

What is a Keto Diet?

WHY IT WORKS

The Keto Diet is an eating plan with high fat, moderate protein and low carbohydrate. It ends the rollercoaster of spikes and crashes of blood sugar, which allows the body to burn fat. There are many variations of low carb diets. The Keto Diet is one of the most popular low carb style diets with additional features.

Depending on your insulin tolerance and activity level, the number of carbohydrates you take in on a Keto Diet varies. On average, to stay in ketosis one must consume not more than 50 grams of carbs per day. Others need to keep carb consumption to somewhere between 20-50 grams per day. Your number may 50 or somewhere lower, but probably won't be higher than 50 grams and not lower than 20 grams

The Ketogenic Diet or Keto Diet is a particular form of low carb diet, with intention of obtaining a specific ratio of macronutrients or macros in the body and to maintain ketosis. Fat, protein and carbohydrates are macronutrients. The Ketogenic Diet is normally 70% fat, 25% protein and 5% carbohydrates.

In general, the Keto Diet is very low in carbohydrates, high in fat and medium in protein.

Don't let this formula scare you. You will feel full and satisfied on this diet, and it will become second nature as you learn and implement it in your lifestyle. It's really very simple.

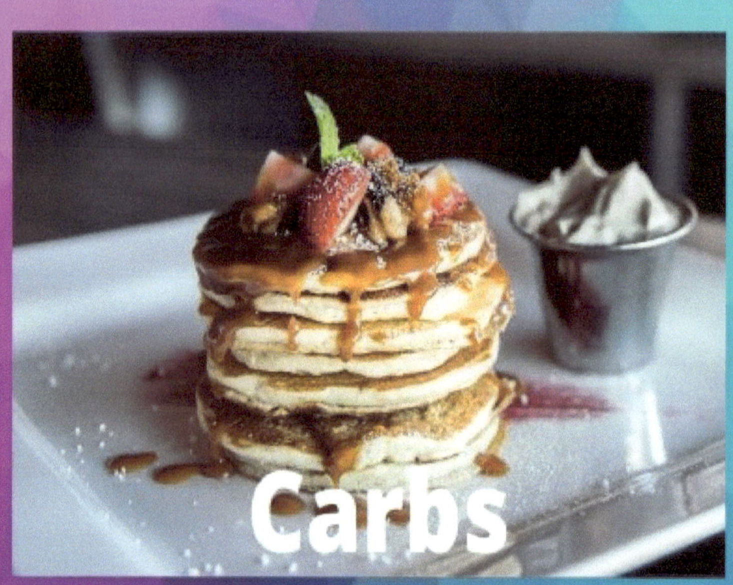

The most crucial factor in achieving ketosis is eating a very low-carbohydrate diet.

Your body cells usually burn glucose or sugar as their principal fuel source. Most cells can, however, use other fuels like fatty acids and ketones, also known as ketone bodies.

The body holds glucose in the form of glycogen. Glycogen storage is reduced. Hormone insulin levels decline when carb intake is very low. This allows release of fatty acids from your body's fatty stores.

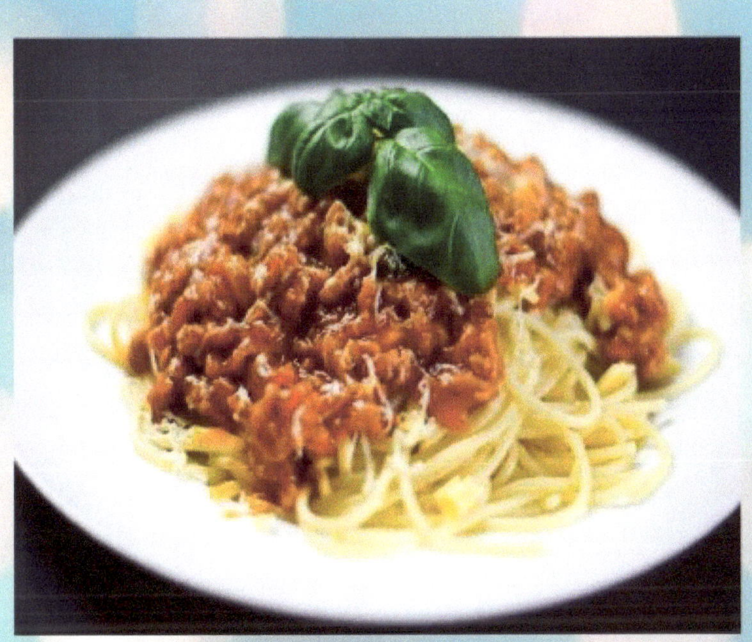

Some fatty acids in your liver are converted to ketones, acetone and beta-hydroxybutyrate. Sections of the brain use ketones as a source of energy.

Carb restriction to induce ketosis varies by individuals. Many people can achieve ketosis with net carbohydrates of 20 grams a day. Others can reach ketosis by consuming twice or more. The range is generally between 20-50 grams per day in order for most people to achieve ketosis.

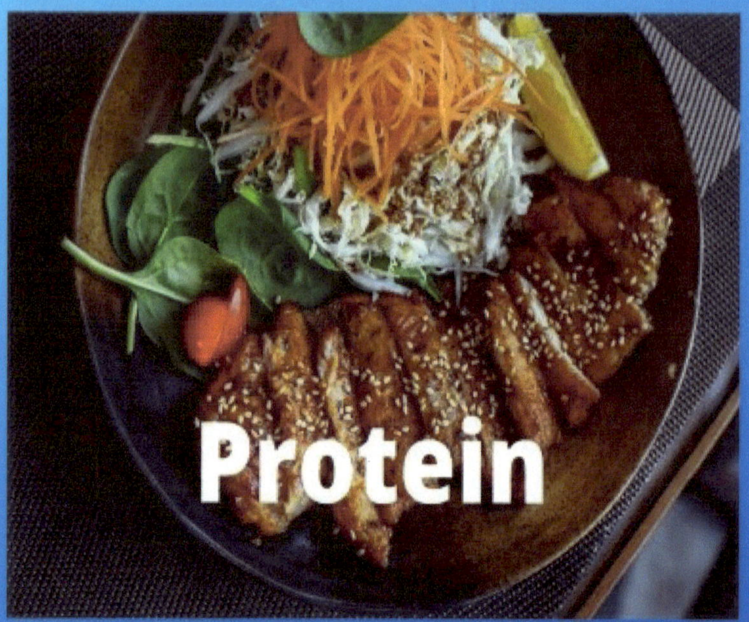

Maintain enough protein consumption. Achieving ketosis requires an adequate but not excessive intake of protein.

Ketogenic Diets lead to increased intake of protein, which provides numerous weight loss benefits, and restricts intake of carbahydrates. This substantially decreases calorie intake, which is necessary for weight loss without counting calories.

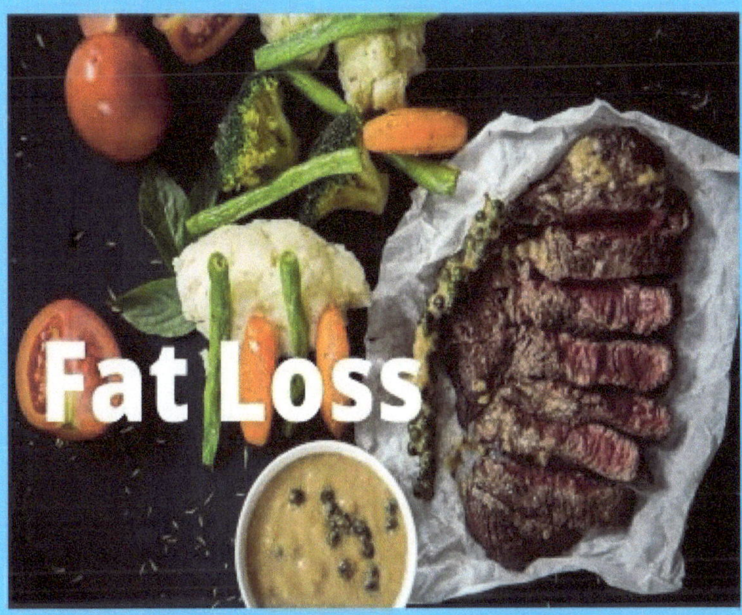

Your abdominal cavity produces a higher proportion of fat loss with help of a Keto Diet. Not all fat is the same in your body. When fat is processed, it determines how it impacts your health and disease risk.

The two main types are subcutaneous fat under your skin and visceral fat accumulated in your abdominal cavity. Visceral fat sits around the liver. Excess visceral fat is linked to inflammation and resistance to insulin—and can cause today's western metabolic dysfunction. Low-carb diets reduce this harmful abdominal fat extremely efficiently.

"You'll feel full and satisfied."

Fats replace the bulk of carbohydrates and provide about 75% of daily calorie consumption. Proteins can account for about 20% of energy needs, while carbohydrates are generally restricted to 5%. A decrease of carbs causes the body to burn fat rather than glucose, a mechanism known as ketosis, using fats as the primary source of energy.

The Ketogenic Diet can help you reach your goal. As you hit that number on the scale you've been searching for, carb consumption can be increased to a level where you can stay in a maintenance state. In maintenance carbohydrates are usually limited to less than 50 grams a day, allowing the process to maintain your goal weight.

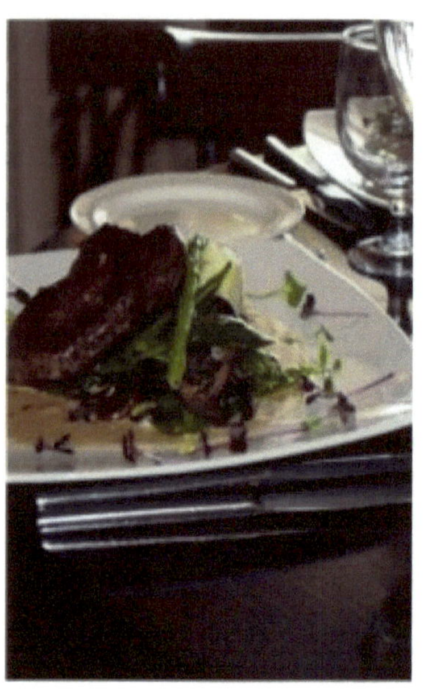

Just Do It!

We hear this question almost daily. A change in lifestyle can be profoundly overwhelming, and people are often confused with contradictory details they don't know where to begin. It's simple.

Just do it!

Don't look back. Do it. Every moment you postpone your journey to start another day, it puts your health at risk. Jump in. Start.

Dedicate yourself to the process, and you are one step closer to your goal weight. Like any change, in the beginning, it takes time and planning. You will learn as you go and it will become second-nature.

You're Ready!

This is one of most significant aspects of starting any diet plan. Wrap your mind around changes you must make and possible setbacks you might experience. Many self-recognized experts with the Keto Diet offer different advice and 'keto rules.' This can confuse and frustrate you.

Stop reading. Get started.

Go through the house and remove high carb foods that might tempt you. Purchase fresh keto foods. Select options easy to prepare that will satisfy your taste buds, so you are less tempted to cheat. This diet allows for plenty of tummy satisfying options, so you should not go hungry.

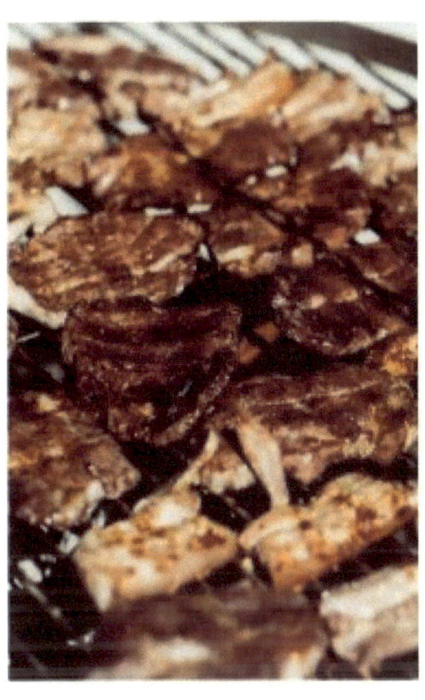

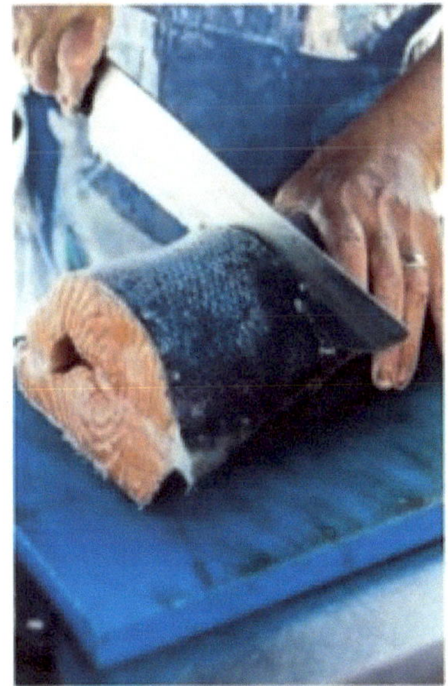

Simple Steps

Follow these basic rules:
A. Eliminate carbs: Check food labels and consume no more than 50g of carbs or less per day.
B. Purchasestaples of your diet: Meat, cheese, eggs, nuts, oils, avocados, oily fish and cream.
C. Eat low--carb vegetables: Fat sources are high in calories. Fill your plate with low-carb vegetables.
D. Experiment: A Ketogenic Diet can be exciting and delicious. You can make ketogenic pasta, brownies, muffins, pudding, ice cream, etc. Try the recipes in this book. Experiment with keto recipes and find those you enjoy.
E. Create a plan before leaving home: When you go out, it can be difficult to find low-carb meals. As with any diet, a strategy and snacks or easily accessible food are essential. Be prepared. Check the restaurant's menu for options before you go, if possible.

Stay on Track

F. Eat what you love: Eating keto friendly foods you love will allow you to stay on track. Treat yourself well. There are fabulous, delectable foods at your disposal.

G. Track progress: As you begin, take photos. Keep records. Calculate and track your weight every three-to-four weeks. You should see visible signs in the way clothing fits. Keeping records allows you reason to celebrate successes, which helps you stay on track. It also allows you to see when you've gone off course and need to make changes to get back on your plan. If improvement stops, reduce portion sizes slightly.

H. Replace minerals: Ketosis changes your body's balance of fluid and minerals. Salt food to minimize changes. You may choose to supplements to help.

I. Add supplements: Ketone salt supplements, MCT oil (5-10 grams twice a day) or cocoa oil daily can be used to improve the ketogenic process. Adding collagen has major benefits to the body.

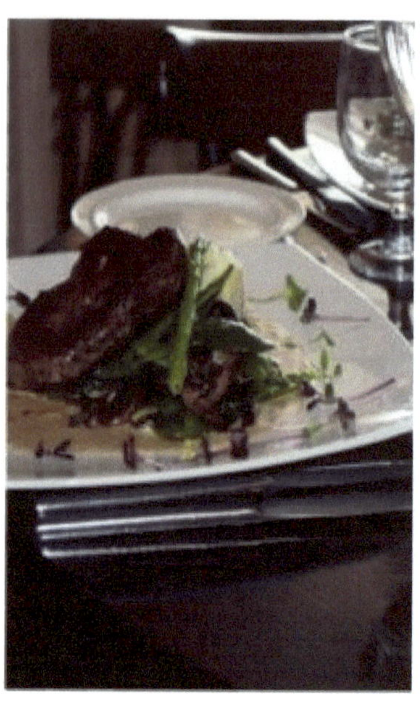

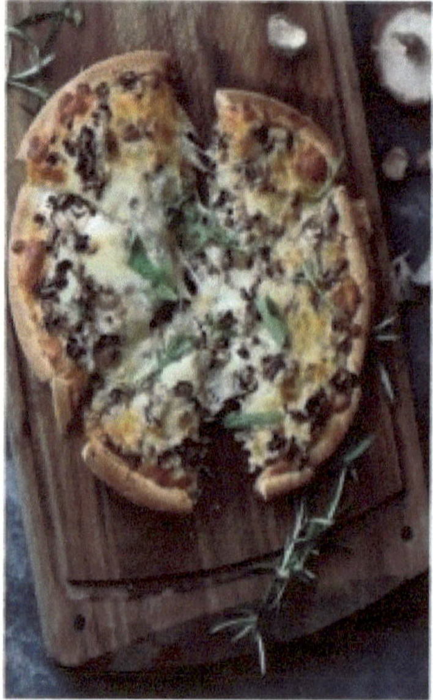

Key to Success

J. Monitor ketone levels: You may want to monitor ketone levels in your urine or blood, as these let you know if carb levels are low enough to produce ketosis. On the basis of current research, laboratory studies show in continuous client testing, nutritional ketosis is achieved at sufficient levels at over 0.5-1.0 mmol / l.

K. Consistency: There is no shortcut to success. Consistency is the most critical factor in any diet, especially the Keto Diet. There are three reasons to be consistent..

1. Consistency helps achieve ketosis.
2. It helps you get past any temporary symptoms the diet change may cause.
3. Increasing consumption of fats and continuing eating high carbs, may cause weight gain instead of loss. You do not want to produce a negative effect.

Keto Diet Meal Plan

If it seems overwhelming to switch to a Ketogenic Diet, don't fret. It doesn't have to be hard. Your emphasis should be on three things.

1) Reduce carbohydrate intake.
2) Increase fat intake.
3) Eat quality protein.

If you do these three simple things consistently, this plan becomes automatic. Carbs must be restricted in order to reach and remain in a ketosis state. Some people can achieve ketosis at 50 grams. Others require less. Some may require only by eating 20 grams of carbohydrates per day to achieve a ketosis state. The lower your intake of carbohydrates, the easier it is to reach and remain in ketosis.

DRINK THESE

Water, sparkling water, green tea, coffee, Certain Alcohol: Alcohol should be limited; however, it is perfectly safe to drink low-carb beverages such as vodka or tequila combined with soda water.

EAT THESE:

Meat: Steak, red meat, bacon, ham, turkey and chicken
Fatty Fish: tuna, mackerel, salmon and trout
Eggs: omega-3 whole eggs
Butter and Cream
Cheese: unprocessed cheeses such as cheddar, goat, cream, blue or mozzarella
Nuts and Seeds: almonds, walnuts, flax seeds, squash seeds, chia, etc.
Oils: extra virgin olive oil, coconut and avocado oil Avocados: whole avocado or fresh guacamole
Low Carb Veggies: most green vegetables
Condiments: salt, pepper, herbs and spices

AVOID THESE:

Processed Sweets: Cake, ice cream, candy, soda, fruit juice
Grains& / Starches: cereal, pasta, rice, wheat-based foods
Fruit: all except small portions of berries
Beans: peas, beans, legumes and lentils Root Vegetables: potatoes, carrots, etc.
Packaged Foods
Alcohol
Sugar-Free Diet Foods

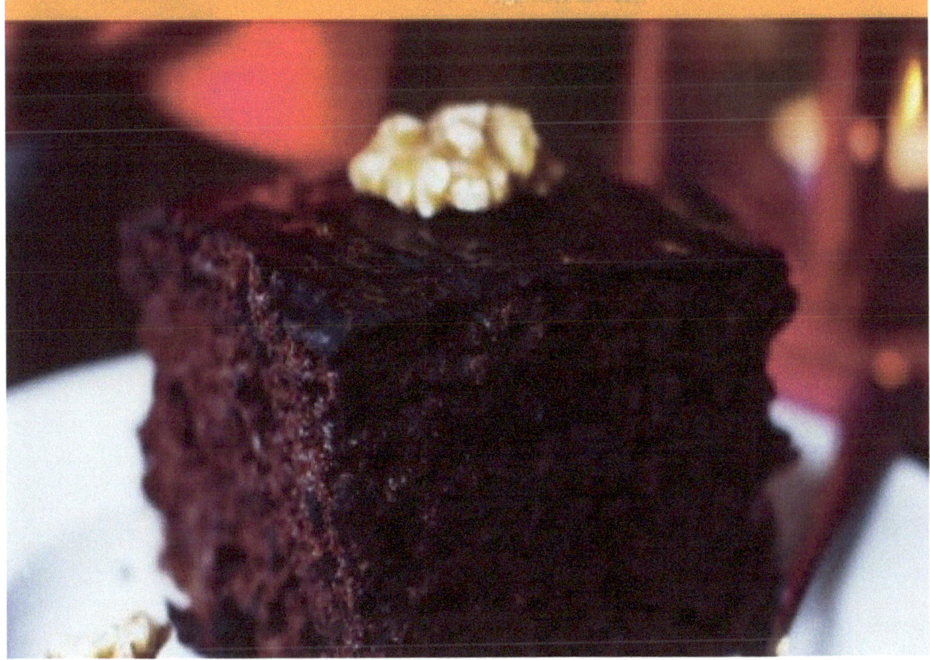

The Easiest Fastest way to "Hack" the Keto Diet?

No guesswork, Research, Or Planning . . .   Just Follow This Link To Make Keto Simple & Fun . . . And Be Shocked At Your Before & After!

Let me show you the easiest, fastest way to hack the keto diet you'll ever find. The Keto diet has been called a "miracle cure all"... because of the diet's benefits. Excess fat (especially around the belly) quickly melting off...... Gaining a ton more energy that most adults forget is even possible......All while eating more delicious foods than ever before......Without suffering from constant hunger......And without craving sugar, or other unhealthy foods like with most diets.

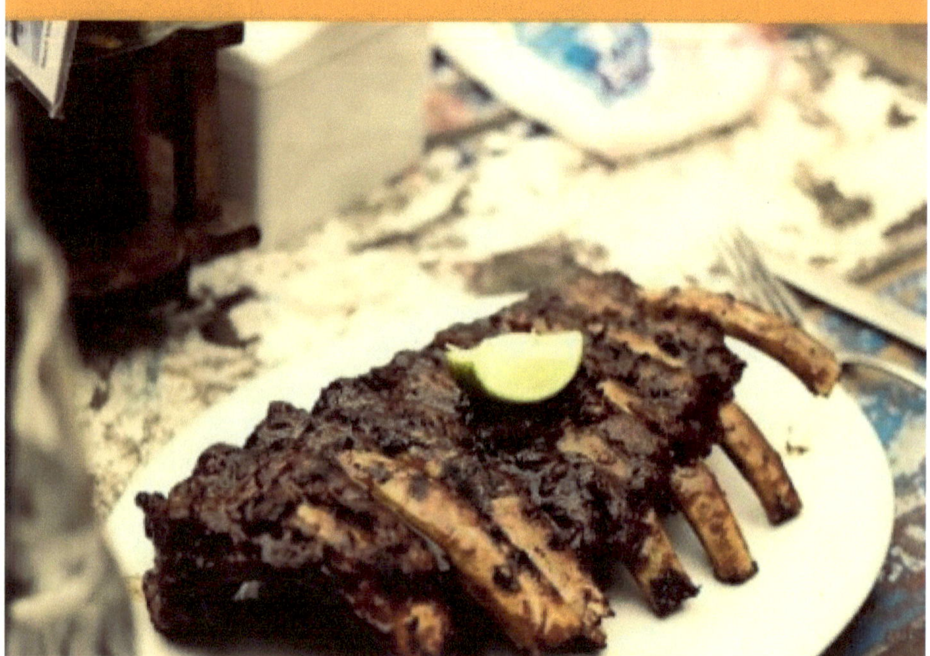

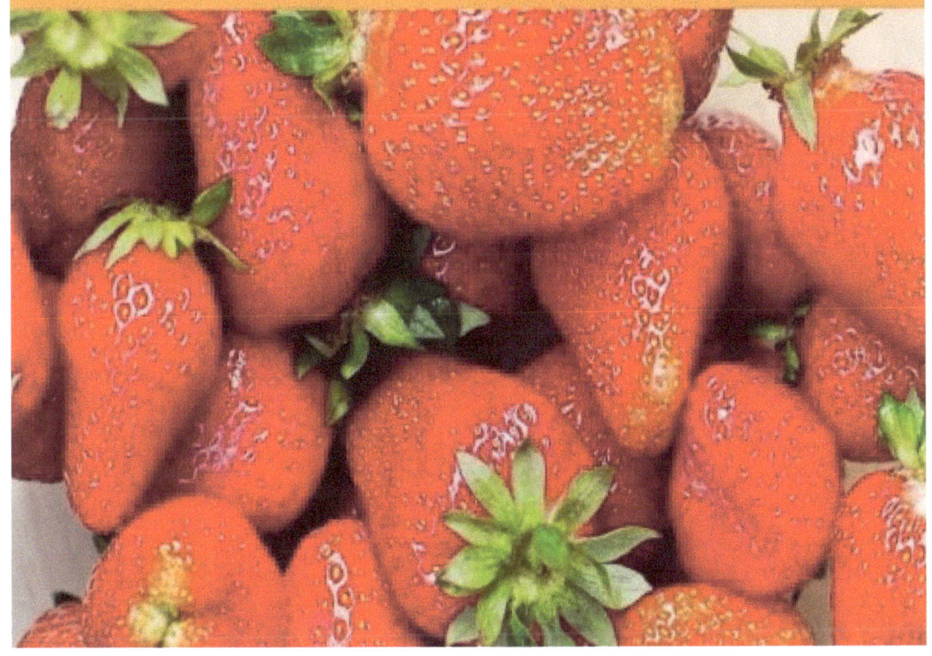

The Easiest, Fastest Way to HACK Keto

THIS is the easiest, fastest way to hack the keto diet you'll ever find. The Keto diet has been called a "miracle cure all".

All because of the ketogenic diet's benefits:
.. Excess fat (especially around the belly) quickly melting off...
.. Gaining a ton more energy that most adults forget is possible.
.. All while eating more delicious foods than ever before...
.. Without suffering from constant hunger.
.. And without craving sugar, or other unhealthy foods like with most diets.

Thousands of people, including celebrities like Gywnneth Paltrow, Halle Berry, Kourtney and Kim Kardashian, and Megan Fox, swear by the benefits of the Keto diet.

Ordinary women, even moms of four kids are seeing themselves shocked at their before and after pictures. Fitting into jeans they haven't worn in decades, and having their doctors shocked at their new healthy numbers.

And that's because the keto diet puts your body into a state of ketosis.
This means your body uses its own fat as fuel.
Most people have their bodies programmed to use sugar as fuel.

But when you're in ketosis and your body uses fat for fuel, that's when you can experience:

All-day, beaming energy. Your mood and happiness bouncing back up. Clearer, smoother skin. Snapping out of brain and mental fogginess. Excess weight practically melting off your trouble areas. Your libido reawakening, roaring back to life.

The problem is, Keto can get complicated quickly. People don't know what to eat on keto. If done incorrectly, they can stall and get discouraged. And they can be overwhelmed by the calculations.

But now, that all changes.

Click here for the easiest, fastest way to "hack" keto.

You'll be looking back at a brand new healthy you before you know it!
Cheers,
LYNDI KAE
SWEETWATER PUBLISHING COMPANY

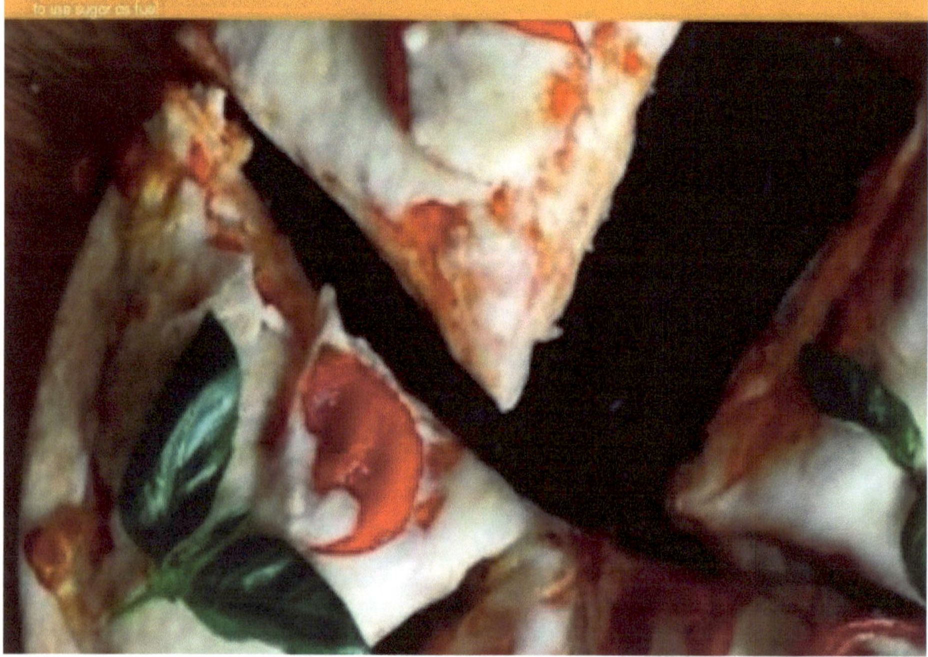

ABOUT THE AUTHOR

Lyndi Kae

Lyndi Kae is an award-winning author with over thirty-six years' experience in research and study of nutrition. She brings to you an easy, step-by-step program to achieve success in the simple Easy Keto Diet program. Easy Keto Guide, Easy Keto Diet, 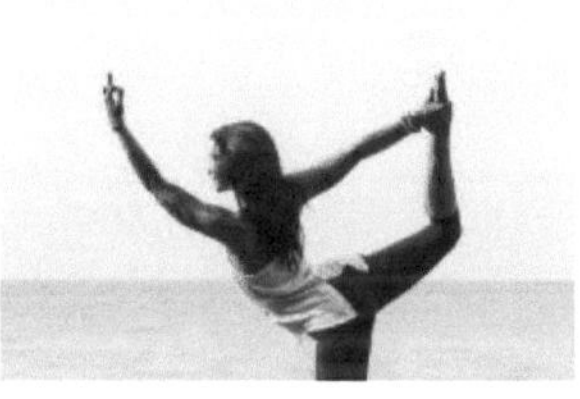 Easy Keto Cooking, Easy Keto Desserts, Easy Keto Journal, Easy Keto Cheat Sheet, Easy Keto Shopping, Easy Keto 7 Day Meal Planner, Easy Keto Cheat Sheet.

Lyndi Kae brings you benefit of over 36 years' research and study of the diet and nutrition industry. Enjoy and be sure to check out the other books in the series.

Also By Lyndi Kae are:

Easy Keto Diet

Easy Keto Cooking

Easy Keto Desserts

Easy Keto Journal

Easy Keto Guide

Easy Keto Cheat Sheet

Easy Keto Shopping Tool

Easy Keto 7 Day Meal Planner

Get them all in a Kit and SAVE! For a great DEAL on the complete KIT through Amazon, contact the publisher.

lyndareesauthor@gmail.com

BOOKS BY THIS AUTHOR

Easy Keteo Guide

This handy guidebook will help you understand how the KETO diet works, science behind it and benefits of the program, so you can determine if the KETO way of life is for you. NO counting calories. Simply stick to this fabulous, healthy eating process while enjoying nutritious, satisfying meals that fuel your body and increase your energy levels. Lose body fat and weight, and improve your health, vitality and focus, while enjoying nutritious protein and fat to help you feel amazing. Life changing eating doesn't have to be difficult.

Easy Keto Diet

Turn your body into a fat burning machine with this step-by-step Easy Keto Diet instruction book. Also look for Easy Keto Cooking, Easy Keto Desserts, and other toolsto help you achieve ketosis, improve your health and appearance, increase energy and get to your ideal weight - Quick!

Easy Keto Cooking

Fabulous, easy recipes filled with antioxidants and healthy fat to improve focus and help you feel free and amazing. This cookbook is a simple tool to help you stick to and enjoy your ketogenic diet.

Life changing eating doesn't have to be difficult.

Easy Keto Desserts

These mouthwatering, simple recipes will keep your sweet tooth happy. They're so deliciously decadent you'll wonder why you didn't go Keto sooner. Fabulous, easy recipes filled with antioxidants and healthy fat to improve focus and help you feel free and amazing. This cookbook is a simple tool to help you stick to and enjoy your ketogenic diet. Life changing eating doesn't have to be difficult.

Easy Keto Journal

This handy journal book will help you keep track of your progress as you enjoy your KETO diet program. NO counting calories. Simply keep track to measure what works. This too pinpoints what adjustments might make it easier to stick to this fabulous, healthy eating program. It also shows you when you have the right to Celebrate Milestones.

Lose body fat and weight, and improve your health and focus, while enjoying nutritious protein and fat to help you feel amazing. This simple tool assists you stick to and enjoy your ketogenic lifestyle. Life changing eating doesn't have to be difficult.

Easy Keto Shopping

This reusable laminated shopping list enables you to breeze through shopping and select nutritious protein, fat and other delicious items without having to think about it much. This time-saving device makes your life so much easier. Life changing eating doesn't have to be difficult.

Easy Keto Cheat Sheet

This amazing reusable tool is a quick and dirty lowdown tha helps keep you on track with your Keto diet lifestyle. Using this, eating the ketogenic way will quickly become second nature. Life changing eating doesn't have to be difficult. Let's make it easy together.

Easy Keto 7 Day Meal Planner

This simple to use tool will help you plan meals quickly and easily so you can stay on track with your Keto diet lifestyle and plan shopping trips with a breeze--and it's reusable. Life changing eating isn't difficult. Let's make it easy together.

UNTITLED